Essential Oils Recipes

Essential Oils and Aromatherapy for Weight Loss, Stress Relief and Happiness

DEDICATION

WELCOME TO THE FASCINATING WORLD OF AROMA

Essential oils have made it so **EASY** to ditch the toxins and use natural recipes for cleaning my home and even **DIY** beauty products. I feel **SO** much better knowing I'm not using dangerous chemicals around my family and my pets...

CONTENTS

CHAPTER 1

Overview of Essential Oils

What are Essential Oils?

An essential oili s a concentrated liquid, hydrophobic in nature and contains aroma compounds from plants. These are also known under the name of volatile oils, ethereal oils, aetherolea, or simply as the "oil of" the particular plant from which they were extracted, such as clove oil. The oil is named as "essential oil" in because it contains the essence of the plant's fragrance from which they have been extracted and they also contain important ingredients that are necessary for one's body.

They are generally extracted by the process of distillation or sometimes by solvent extraction using steam. Essential oils can be used in cosmetics, scents, soaps and other ingredients so as to add flavor and scent. Cleaning products might also be made using essential oils.

Use of Essential Oils

Use of these oils in medicine dates back to prehistoric times. Applications of these oils in medicine are evident through their use as health toners and effective detoxifying agents.

Use of essential oils is declined in scientifically proof-based medicine. Essential oils are helpful in igniting the senses and brightening our spirit. Botanical essences are packed inside the essential oils and help you to discover rich therapeutic potential that cannot be found anywhere else. A solitary oil as well as oils in a blended recipe is enough to promote clarity of mind and hormonal balance. Invigorate your body senses and brighten your day with specially formulated. Essential oil recipes are right for you to take you to a rollercoaster of health. You can use them anytime and anywhere. You can bring the pure essence these oils to your life to help you in leading a young healthy one. Take the medicine to a whole new level. Use them in your massage oils and give yourself the power to restore a sense of balance to your body and spirit. Bring your essential oils experience into full balance. Have you ever imagined how an essence of oil can brighten your day start imagining from today and transform yourself into a new energetic healthy being who can perform daily chores with new zeal and zest and who knows how to keep loved ones happy with themselves. ESSENTIAL OILS are your key to fulfilling and balanced emotional and physical aspects of life.

ESSENTIAL OILS also help you to rediscover peace, joy and balance in everyday life. Use them for diffusion, baths, massage, inhalation, or topical application.

CHAPTER 2

Aromatherapy

What is Aromatherapy?

Aromatherapy, also known as essential oil therapy, can be defined as the art and science of using plant material and aromatic plant oils, especially essential oils, for the purpose of altering one's mood, cognitive, psychological or physical wellbeing.

The inhaled aroma from these essential oils is widely used to stimulate brain function. Essential oils can also be absorbed through the skin, from where they proceed through one's bloodstream and eventually leads to whole-body healing and relief. Whether inhaled or applied on the skin, essential oils are gaining attention as an alternative treatment for stress, infections and various health problems.

Aroma Therapist

Aroma therapists, who specialize in the art of aromatherapy, use blends of curative essential oils which can be supplied through topical application, inhalation, massage or water immersion to stimulate a desired response.

General Benefits

Numerous benefits attach themselves to aromatherapy in the long run. One's mood enhances and a general feeling of well-being courses through one's mind. It improves blood and lymphatic circulation through massage and the use of essential oils. It's the best tool in eradicating anxiety as according to a community survey, aromatherapy embraces hundred percent success rate. It plays a role in soothing the nerves and elevating your emotions, taking you out of the darkness of depression and restlessness. It reduces *Alopecia areata* (hair loss). With abdominal massage using aromatherapy, constipation can be relieved. Studies have found that people suffering from rheumatoid arthritis, cancer and headaches require fewer pain medications when they take to aromatherapy. Moreover it can be used to eliminate itching, a common side-effect for those receiving dialysis.

What is the history of Aromatherapy?

Aromatherapy has been used for remedial purposes for about 6000 years. The ancient Chinese, Egyptians, Indians, Greeks and Romans used essential oils in medicines, drugs, perfumes and cosmetics. Moreover, they were also commonly used for spiritual and ritualistic purposes. Rene-Maurice Gattefosse, a French chemist, discovered the properties of lavender oil. He used lavender oil on a burn he got from an explosion in his laboratory. Afterwards, he unleashed how lavender oil can be used for treating burns, skin infections, gangrene and wounds in soldiers during World War I. He founded the science of aromatherapy. Later on, massage therapists, beauticians, nursed, physiotherapists, doctors and other health care providers started using aromatherapy. Today, many lotions, candles and beauty products are being sold as aromatherapy, though many of these products might contain synthetic fragrances which are not as effective as essential oils.

Future of Aromatherapy

The world of Aromatherapy evolves as the science progresses. The ancient methods now merged with modern science to elevate its efficacy.

Today, the emerging model_ evidence-based aromatherapy_ affiliate the best of all models (The British Model, the French Model, and to a lesser extent the German Model) and enriches them with scientific evidence. In this way the art of aromatherapy embraces efficiency and becomes a promising alternative therapy.

Fill Sunrik

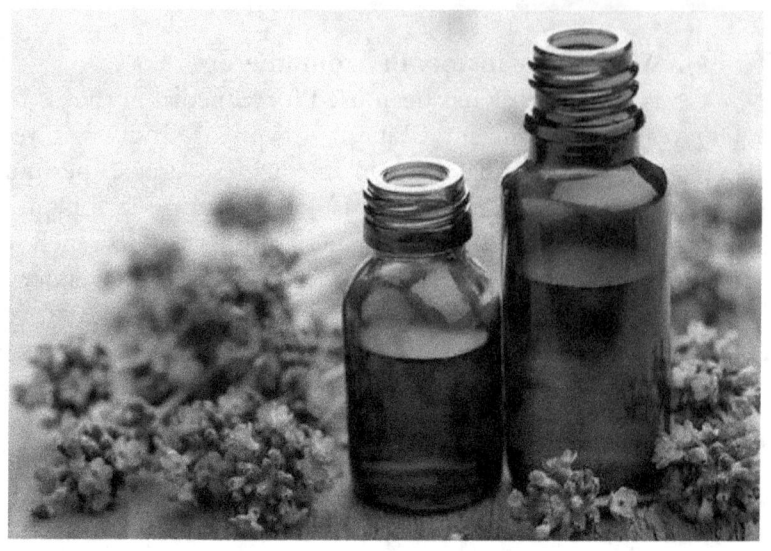

CHAPTER 3

Importance of Essential Oils

Women have been using essential oils since ancient times to preserve their beauty. In addition to being used for enhancing beauty, all essential oils also offer therapeutic effects on the skin as well as influence the state of mind. Therefore, by applying them, you care not only about beauty, but also about mood.

Names and Modes of Actions of Essential Oils

There are a few essential oils which have marvelous properties and functions. These essential oils are as under:

NAME OF OIL	*FUNCTIONS*
ORANGE	Relieves headaches, muscle pain, joint pain, neuralgia, and menstrual pain. It helps to get rid of anxiety and insomnia. Do not apply the essential oil of orange skin in the sun.
ROSES	Moisturizes and strengthens skin,

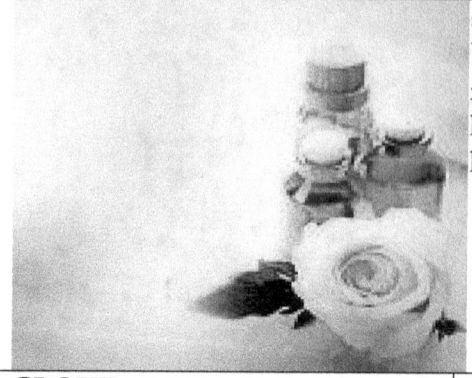

smooth out wrinkles. Using as massage oil relieves stress. Also helps with acne and herpes.

CLOVE

Acts as an anti-inflammatory agent. Baths with the addition of a few drops of this oil aid to restore lost strength from physical exhaustion.

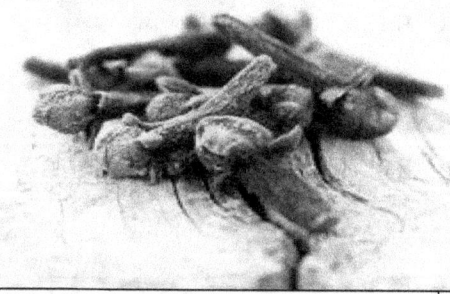

GRAPEFRUIT

Offers cleansing and refreshing, properties. Helps to restore natural secretion of the sebaceous glands in particular. Also aids in strengthening the nervous system, relieving anxiety, irritation and normalizing the liver functions.

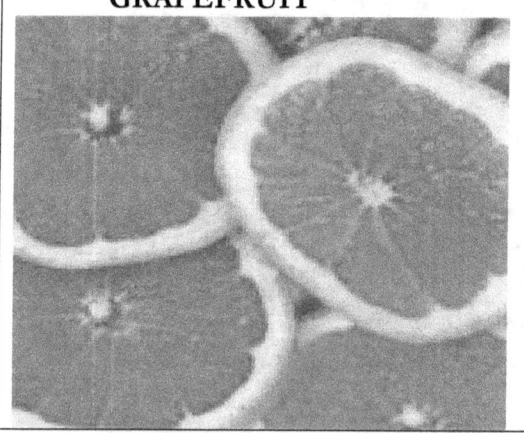

SANDAL

Brightens the skin, and helps eliminating acne. Effective with itchy skin and wrinkles.

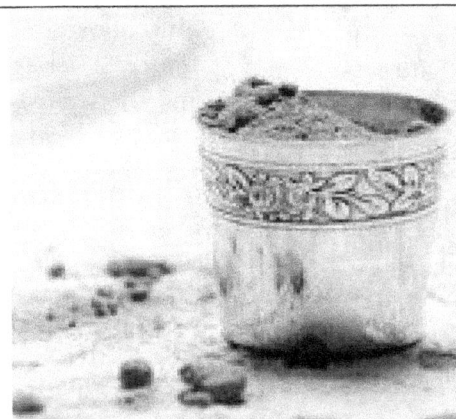	Helps in eliminating insomnia and stress. It is used in the treatment of sore throat and runny nose
LAVENDER 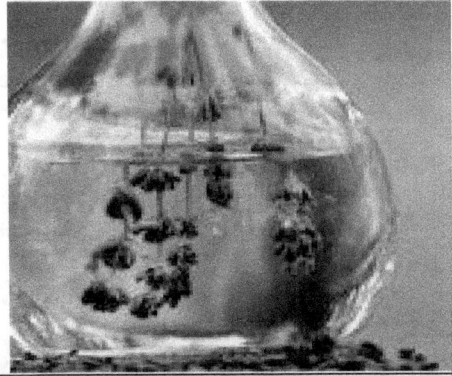	Eliminates insomnia and tearfulness. It has deodorant, anti-inflammatory antiseptic properties. It is useful for every skin type.
PEPPERMINT 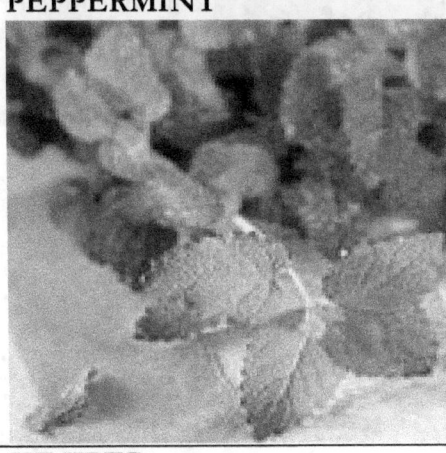	Has antiseptic and stimulating effect. Awakens the skin, and helps relief bad sleep. It is used in disorders of the digestive system, as well as viral diseases and colds. It also speeds up recovery from sunburn.
JUNIPER	Enhances mental activity. It has anti-inflammatory and

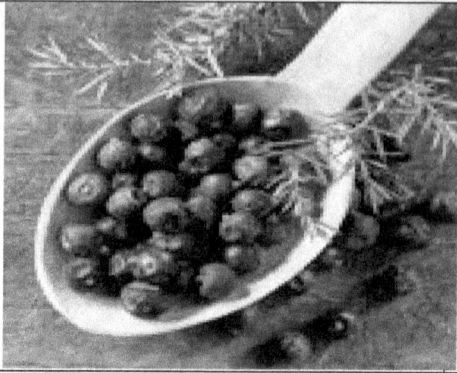	antiseptic properties. It improves elasticity of skin. Effective against irritation and itching from insect bites
ROSEMARY 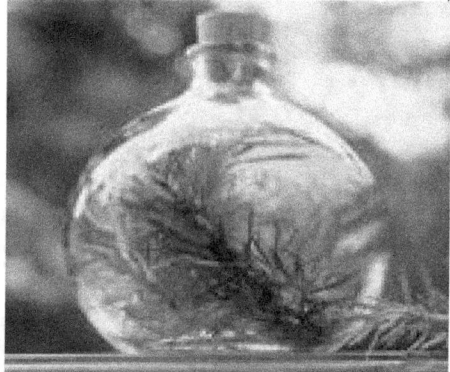	Relieves physical and mental fatigue, apathy. It reduces the secretion of sebum and smooths the skin. Suitable for acne prone skin.
TEA TREE 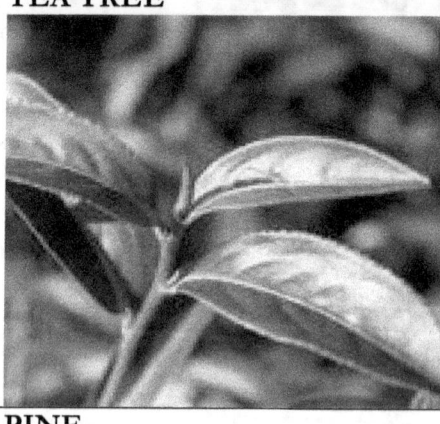	It has powerful anti-inflammatory action and antiseptic. Used against skin lesions, acne, to eliminate unpleasant foot odor, to relieve fatigue, Baths with the addition of tea tree oil help the body recover.
PINE	Tonic, increases stamina and relieves stress. It has antiseptic, anti-inflammatory action. Bath with the

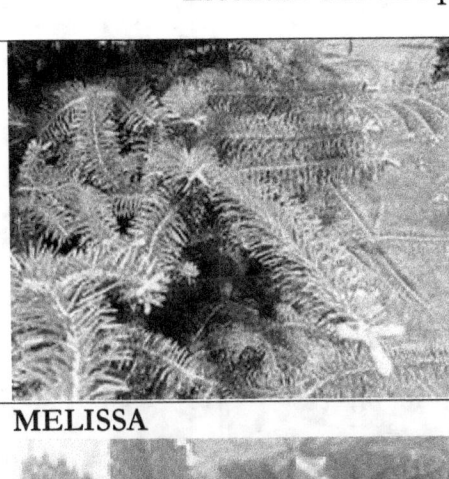

addition of pine oil promotes restoration of forces after nervous and physical exhaustion.

MELISSA

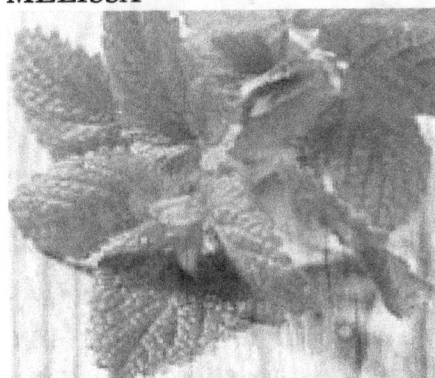

Helps with depression and reducing irritability. Improves memory and adjusts sleep habits. Strengthens the immune responses.

NUTMEG

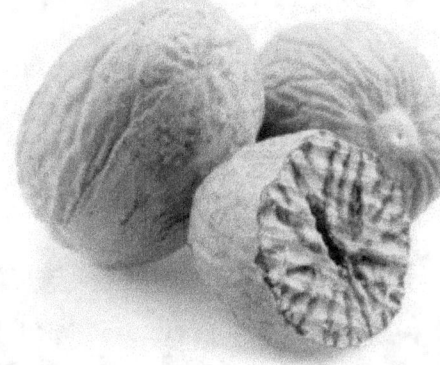

Improves blood circulation and helps improve skin too. Helps fight fungal diseases.

LEMON

Boosts energy and positive emotions. It has antiseptic and deodorizing effect. The perfect remedy for wrinkles. Effective for

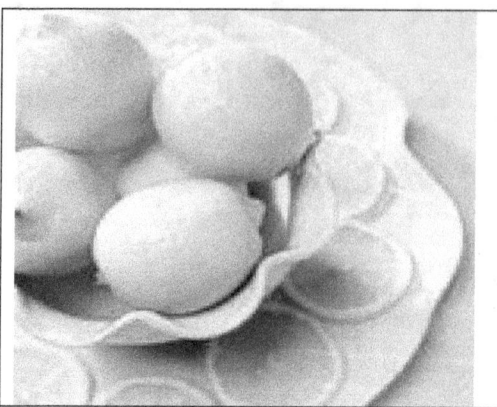

oily skin and hair.

EUCALYPTUS

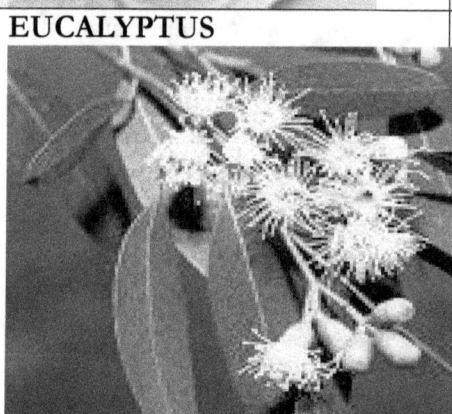

It has antiseptic, anti-herpetic, regenerating and anti-inflammatory action. It is used against cold infections, and runny nose.

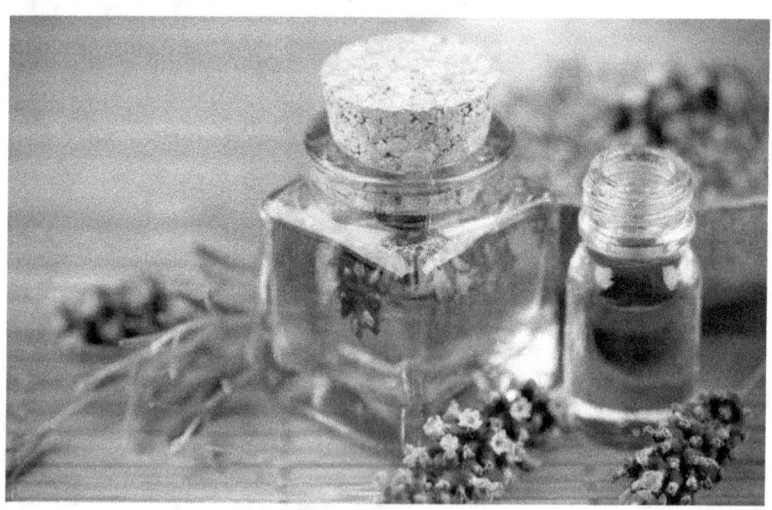

Essential Oils Recipes

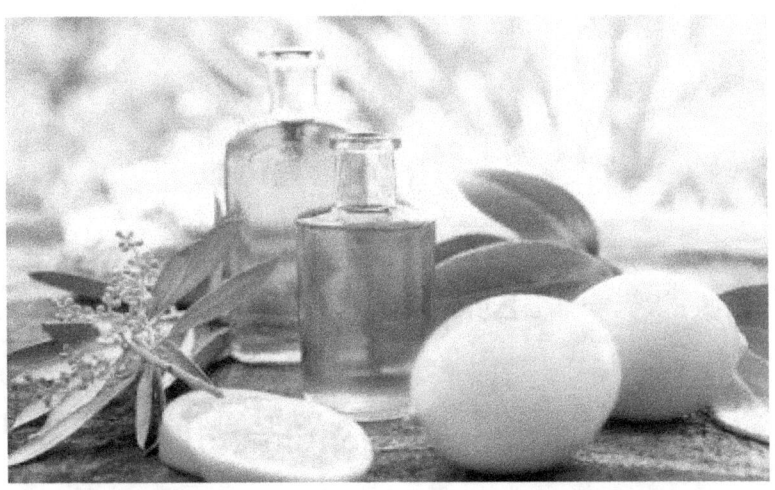

CHAPTER 4

Essential Oil Recipes

How to use Essential Oil Recipes?

The essential oils that you choose will depend upon the purpose. You can make your own essential oils by using the ingredients I have mentioned in this book. Play with your ingredients and use them the way you want to. Keep your book and your ingredients ready and there you go.

Make sure that you pay attention to precautions for each oil and method of application. If you have allergy with certain ingredients, make sure you don't use them in making your oils. Dilution is a very important factor in making the oils. Make sure you dilute your oils properly to get the best out of your favorite ingredients. Diluting your oils will enhance their detoxification properties to the maximum.

Different Methods of Using Essential Oils

Essential oils may be:

applied to the skin

inhaled

ingested

Choosing the application method:

The chosen method of application depends upon the results you are expecting. Some oils might be irritating to the skin but would do ok when ingested. If you have a wound you would want to go for tropical application but in case you want to see long lasting effects against anti-aging, you would definitely ingest your oils. Mood affects can be altered by inhalation and inhalation method is preferred in case of fast effects.

Inhaling Essential Oils

This can be done by techniques listed as under:

Diffuser: Oils are placed with water in the device. Diffuser would not burn them but heat them so they evaporate. Make sure you read all the instructions before using the diffuser.

Dry Evaporation: In this method essential oils can be placed on a cotton ball or tissue and allowed to evaporate into the air. You may also sniff the cotton ball.

Steam: Drops of essential oil are poured in the steaming water and the oils are inhaled.

Spray: Drops of essential oils can be used along with water so as to use them in the form of inhaler.

How do I Apply Essential Oils Topically?

Essential oils should NOT be directly applied to skin and even if they need to be they should be properly diluted to 3%. For massage use 1% percent diluted solution and for toddlers, the concentration of essential oils should not be more that 0.25%.

Dilutions can be made in the carrier oils and these carrier oils are available in the store. Examples are sweet almond oil, apricot kernel oil, grape seed oil, jojoba oil, or avocado oil. These oils do not have a strong smell of their own and their aroma can be easily masked by the essential oil ingredients.

Anti-microbial may also be added so as to speed up the process of wound healing.

They may be applied:

directly to skin

Gargle

Bath

Massage

5. Ingesting the Essential Oils

Essential oils may also be ingested with green tea and other beverages.

Fill Sunrik

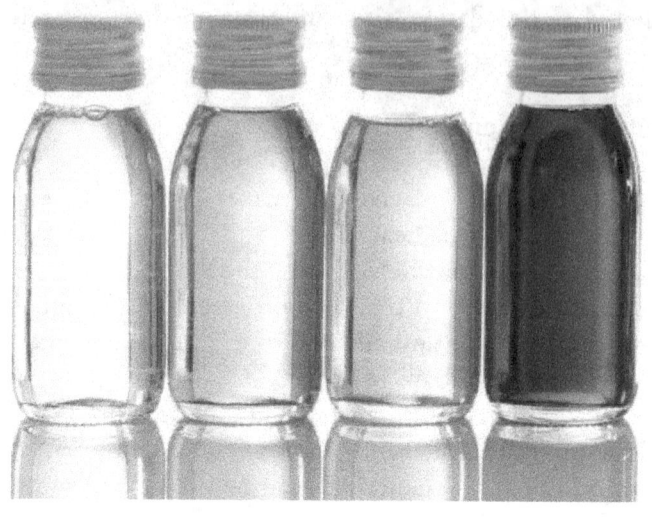

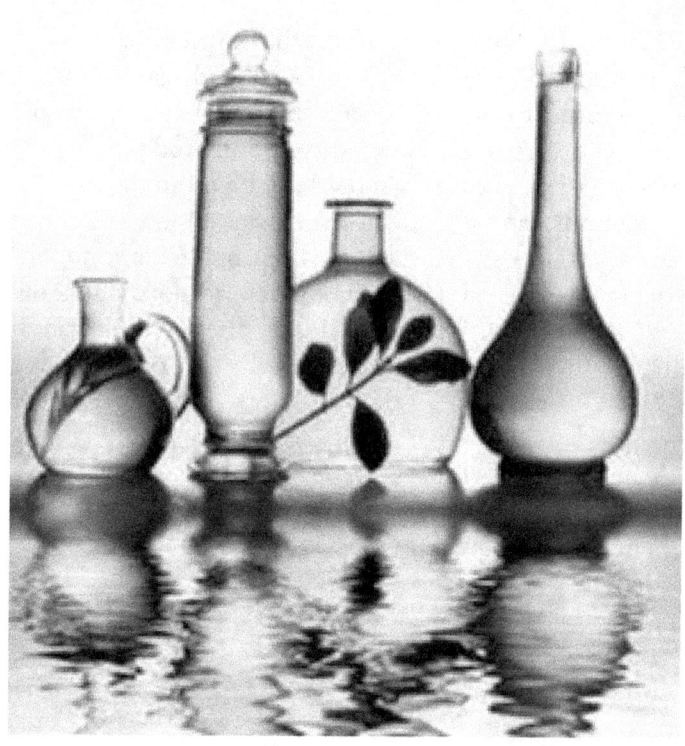

CHAPTER 5

Benefits of Essential Oils

The benefits of using essential oils are vast and diverse. We as humans are dependent upon plants in one way or the other. A broad variety of plants is used in our daily life for oxygen, clothing, building, and bringing harmony and balance to our lives. There are many qualities of plants that make them useful one way or other. The extracts of plant leaves, flowers, roots, or bark are incredible tools for us to use in our everyday lives, and when we are facing serious problems and looking for healthy solutions.

Essential oils definitely carry the essence of the plants in such a proper quantity and potent form that a single drop of essential oils is equally good as multiple teaspoons of herbs. They can be applied in a multiple different ways to make them useful and effective.

Most of the essential oils have **antibacterial, antimicrobial, antiviral, anti-inflammatory, antiseptic, and antibiotic properties that are rendered to the useful ingredients present in them**. In addition to these qualities, essential oils can also be used against ailments like diarrhea, asthma, colic, Cold, Tension, tuberculosis, Skin issues, inflammation, insomnia, stress, infections, insomnia, low libido, mold, Hot flashes, hormone imbalances, Candida, detoxifying, tumors, Muscular pain, cartilage damage, digestive problems, blackheads, Bone spurs, carpal tunnel and varicose veins.

Beside these impressive qualities, they are used for transferring very pleasurable sensory experiences within seconds because of the fragrances and refreshing natures. Essential oils are also used for enhancing beauty and they have been used for the purpose for centuries. Most beautiful Mughal queens are known to have used aromatized essential oils to keep themselves fresh and graceful.

These are made from distilling or extraction of different parts of plants, including the flowers, leaves, roots, resin and peels. They can also be made by soaking the ingredients together.

We may benefit from their antioxidant, antimicrobial and anti-inflammatory properties. The demand of healing essential oils is growing in popularity as they have proven themselves as natural medicine with no side effects.

We all get excited about scents, but its more exciting to know that scents can actually improve health. Essential oils can be good enough to help you relax and sleep soundly. They also help in improving your skin and the process of digestion. They can heal you mentally, physically as well as emotionally.

You shouldn't apply most oils directly to skin, as the high concentration can cause irritation. Essential oils should be diluted with water or a carrier oil like jojoba or almond the way I have explained in the previous chapter, to get most out of them. About ingesting essential oils, you must first see your doctor or aroma therapist to guide you if a particular essential oil can be ingested or not. But I suggest that even if ingestion is a must you should use little quantity with great amount of beverage.

They aren't technically oils as they lack fatty acids in them. But rather they're highly concentrated extracts of plants. A huge amount of plant can be used to get a little quantity of essential oil but they offer a great deal of benefits no matter how little they are in quantity.

CHAPTER 6

Essential Oils Recipes for Weight loss

Introduction to Weight loss

There are many ways to get rid of extra weight. Most of the weight loss techniques will make you hungry and unsatisfied. If you have willpower, then hunger will cause you give up on your plans to lose weight quickly.

The 3-step plan outlined here will:

Reduce your appetite significantly.

Make you lose weight fast, without being hungry.

Improve your metabolic health at the same time.

All of this is supported by scientific studies.

Magical essential oil recipes for weight loss

1) Aromatherapy for Weight Loss-Mint Power

30 drops Sandal essential oil

10 drops Peppermint essential oil

5 drops Ylang Ylang essential oil

2 drops Mint essential oil

2) Aromatherapy for Weight Loss- Citrus freshness

20 drops Lemon essential oil
30 drops Grapefruit essential oil
10 drops Ylang Ylang essential oil

3)Aromatherapy Weight Loss- Herbal essence
15 drops Eucalyptus essential oil
30 drops Clove essential oil
1 drop Oregano essential oil
1 drop Tea tree essential oil

4) Aromatherapy Weight Loss- Digestive speed up
30 drops Peppermint essential oil
20 drops Pine essential oil
10 drops Lemon essential oil

5) Aromatherapy Weight Loss- No more stress eating
30 drops of Sandalwood essential oil
15 drops of Spearmint essential oil
5 drops of Grape fruit essential oil

CHAPTER 7

Essential Oils Recipes for Stress Relief

Introduction to Stress Relief

For most of us, relaxation means zoning yourself out in front of the TV at the end of a stressful day. But this does little to minimize the damaging effects of stress. To effectively combat stress, we need to activate our body's innate relaxation responses. This can be done by practicing relaxation techniques such as deep breathing, meditation, rhythmic exercise, and yoga regularly. Fitting these activities into your life can help reduce everyday stress and boost your energy and mood and incorporating essential oils will also prove to be excellent enhancers for weight loss.

Essential oils work differently based upon the constituents they contain. Based upon the state of the individual constituents they can be stimulating as well as calming. It's almost like these essential oils are able to "know" what is required. So an agitated patient will find they receive a calming effect from an essential oil, while another patient who might be feeling lethargic may find an energetic effect from the same oil.

Essential oils tend to release others of stress which can be agitation, anger, anxiousness, tension and fear but, given time, an individual can get frustrated and down therefore, the value of essential oils is actually in being able to restore one's balance.

Aromatherapy Recipes for Stress Relief

Below are given magical recipes of essential oils which relieve you of the stress, anxiety, nervousness and depression. You must try them.

#1
30 drops of orange essential oil
10 drops of lavender essential oil
10 drops of rosemary essential oil
1 drop of lemon essential oil

#2
20 drops of pine essential oil
5 drops of nutmeg essential oil
10 drops of rosemary essential oil
1 drop of orange essential oil

#3
30 drops of rose essential oil
10 drops of tea tree essential oil
5 drops of nutmeg essential oil

#4
20 drops of pine essential oil
5 drops of nutmeg essential oil
10 drops of rosemary essential oil
1 drop of orange essential oil
#5
30 drops of lavender essential oil
10 drops of pine essential oil
5 drops of grape fruit essential oil

Essential Oils Recipes

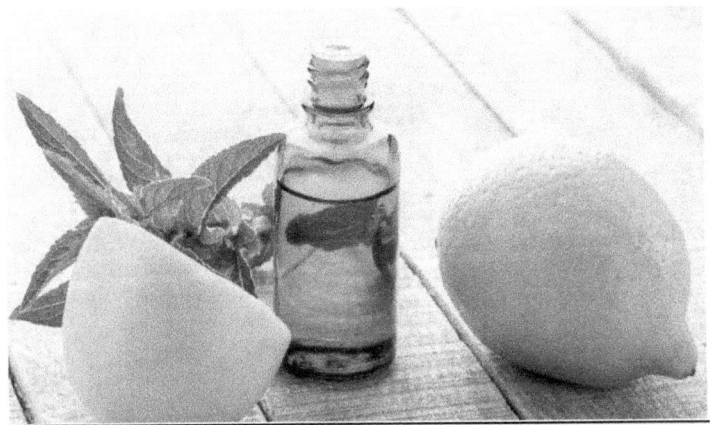

CHAPTER 8

Essential Oils – Way to Happiness

It seems absurd that essential oils make you happy. But, it is true. You can see for yourself.

How can essential oils make you happy?
When you are peaceful and calm from inside, you feel light and everything around you makes you feel relaxed. Essential oils are natural and persuade you to feel nature by smelling deliciously. Essential oils are deprived of additives, cheap alcohols and synthetics, which make you experience the bliss through mother earth.

Essential oils positively enhance and improve moods by affecting different parts of the brain. Hormone production is also affected by essential oils which synthesize a body matching joyous and good feelings. This way, they can change your focus in no time.

The natural scent of essential oils is the carrier of the coded molecules of information, which can transform your brain into a more cohesive and perceptive mind. The magic that is possessed by the energy affects the subtle energies of the body. This, in turn, expands your experience of nature and life and paves the pathway of happiness for you.

2. Recipes of Happy Essential Oils

When you know that the happy essential oils exist, then you must want to know the recipes of these essential oils.

FEEL THE FRAGRANCE
Add 30 drops of oil to an oil burner in the below-mentioned recipes.

Improve your Relations
Orange	9 drops
Geranium	8 drops
Palmarosa	13 drops

Make Yourself Happy
Lemongrass	9 drops
Mandarin	9 drops
Cinnamon	8 drops
Cedarwood Himalayan	4 drops

Release Yourself
Bergamot	10 drops
Juniper	7 drops
Rose Geranium	8 drops
Clary Sage	5 drops

Skin Oil Treatment

To a tablespoon of carrier oil, add one or two drops of essential oil. Oil can be slightly warmed if desired, which can prove to be very relaxing. When you massage your face gently with this oil for 10 minutes, you can feel the real soothing effect of the oils. An oil mask on your face can be covered by a warm or a cool wet facecloth, which acts as a compress over the oil mask. Excess oil can be eliminated from your skin with a cloth or a tissue. Afterwards, you can feel the elimination of all the worries and the empowering of happiness inside you along with the glowing skin.

Olive oil	10 drops
Lavender	3 drops
Geranium	2 drops

Addition of Essential Oil to the bottom of the Shower

Hot water baths make you feel relaxed and fresh. When you take showers, you want to release all your stress and tensions, leaving you with nothing but happiness. You need to put a special essential oil in your bath tub. You will feel out of this world when your whole body will be immersed in that shower containing the essential oil. Do not let the water sink for a few minutes. Now, feel the water, breathe in the medicinal goodness of the oil and feel the happiness proliferating inside your heart.

Petitgrain   5 drops

4. Freshening and Nourishing Body Oil Mix

If you want to keep your body happy along with your mind and heart, then add 3 essential oils to your daily routine.

Rosewood   5 drops
Lemon   4 drops
Basil   2 drop

For proper nourishing of a body, a person needs to smile. Once you smile, your body is relieved from the extra stress.

Pink Grapefruit   5 drops
Jasmine   3 drops

Once you learn to be grateful to others, the feelings of happiness and joy empowers your body and mind. For that, you can rely on two essential oils.

Peru Balsam   5 drops
Lavender   4 drops

Essential Oils Recipes

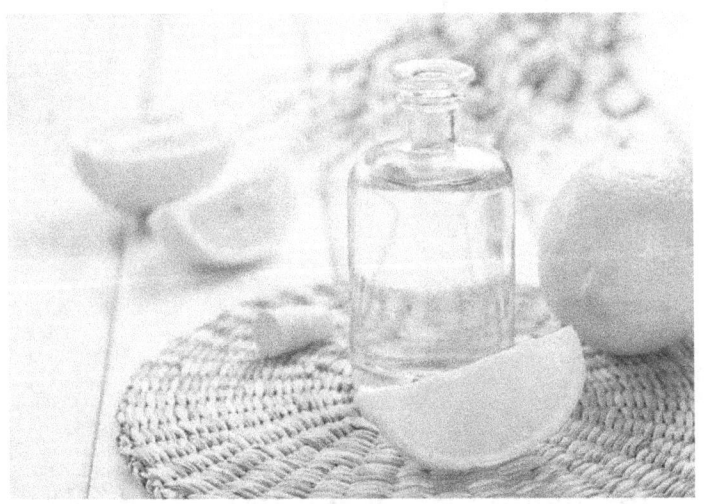

CHAPTER 9

Therapeutic Baths with Monoad Ditives

Using various additives to bath water, it is possible to change the nature of the bath effect. It must ensure to maintain the thermal regime, the duration of the bath and localization effects, that is, those factors that are critical to the overall impact of the bath. Efficiency of bath additives can be manifested in different ways. Mineral vegetable substances may be absorbed either through the skin or through mucosal tunics during respiratory, if these are volatile, aromatic substances. If a focus of disease is located on a body surface, the additives take effect right away and often more surely than at intake. Finally, essential vegetable oils can make the bath more enjoyable. Herbal supplements are used to baths in the form of infusion or decoction of fresh or dried herbs. If you are prone to allergic reactions of the skin, the use of bath additives should be treated with caution.

Baths with monoadditives at various diseases. Hot baths with herbal decoctions are taken 1-3 times a week. The duration of such baths is about 20 minutes. To prepare an herbal bath, pour 3-4 liters of cold water on 1 kg of fresh herbals (unless the amount is not specified in the recipe) and leave it to swell for 1/4 of an hour. Then simmer the mixture for 5 minutes and let it infuse for 10-15 minutes. Strained decoction is added to already prepared bath water.

Essential Oils Recipes

By mixing various herbs, you can create herbal mixtures for baths yourself and achieve the desired effect. The following baths also give a good result at various diseases.

Yeast baths help at skin itching, rubefactions, irritations and other allergic problems on the skin very well. In order to prepare the solution, you need to dissolve 100 g of yeast in 1/2 liter of warm water and to pour it into the bathtub after complete dissolution. The water temperature should be 36-37 °C.

Soda baths help at skin diseases in adults and exudative diathesis in children very well. The water temperature should be 36-37 °C.

Baths of decoction of dried walnut leaves are made at festering rashes, acne. To prepare the decoction, you need to pour 1 liter of warm water on 300 g of the dried ground raw, to boil it for 20 minutes, to let it infuse for 3-4 hours, to strain and to add the concentrated decoction to bath water.

Baths of decoction of oregano help at eczema. To prepare the decoction, you need to pour 3 liters of water on 100 g of crushed dried oregano sprigs and flowers, to boil it for 10 minutes, to strain and to add it to prepared bath water.

A bath with wine vinegar is effective at excessive sweating.

Skin diseases are treated with baths with the addition of decoction of rhizomes of couch-grass. In order to prepare the decoction, you need to pour 10 liters of water on 80 g of the ground raw, to boil it for 30 minutes, to let it infuse for 4 hours, to strain and to add the concentrated decoction to bath water. Baths should be taken daily; the water temperature is 40 °C.

Green tea, added to the bath, provides an excellent therapeutic and cosmetic effect, relieves irritation, soothes the nervous system. To prepare the decoction, you need to pour 10 liters of water on 100 g of the raw, to boil and let it infuse for10 minutes, to strain it and to add the concentrated decoction to bath water. Baths should be taken daily; the water temperature is 36-37 ° C.

A glass of milk powder, added to bath water, has a wonderful soothing effect on the skin, smooths wrinkles.

Rose petals have a rejuvenating effect. Rose essential oil can be added to a bath. It moisturizes dry skin and is great for aging skin.

Half a cup of olive oil, added to bath water, softens and nourish the skin, restoring its smoothness and elasticity.

Coniferous bath relieves fatigue, has a calming effect on the nervous system. Such bath should not be hot. Baths with essential oils of coniferous trees is prescribed to stimulate the metabolic processes in the skin and reduce the excitability of the nervous system. Up to 50 ml of essential oil are added to a bath.

Fragrant baths of decoction of pine needles or of the same essential oil also relieve from a headache. Also, pine needles are suitable for soothing bathing and to relieve from pain in the heart. In order to prepare the decoction, you need to take needles, sprigs, pine cones, to pour with cold water, completely covering them, simmer for half an hour, let it infuse for 12 hours. The decoction should be brown.

Baths of wormwood, taken before going to bed, are used as a sedative, almost sleeping medicine. They can be taken 2-3 times a week before bedtime. A decoction is prepared for baths: 200 g of dry plant is poured by 1 liter of boiling water and left to infuse for an hour in a warm place. The infusion is poured into a prepared bath at a temperature not lower than 37 °C. This bath relieves stress and relaxes. You can take it for up to 20 minutes. It is good to take 10 baths in order to fix the health effect.

Baths of decoction of wild rose roots are recommended at paralysis.

Folk medicine uses baths and hot poultices of fresh young tops and leaves of the vine to treat radiculitis, lumbago and other neurological diseases.

It is necessary to take a therapeutic bath every third day (besides the usual hygiene procedures) for 15-20 minutes at excess weight. The initial water temperature should be 37-38 °C; then, adding hot water, bring the temperature to 41-42 °C. Hot water speeds up metabolism, which promotes weight loss. Baths with the addition of soda help to get rid of fat deposits on the stomach. Bath with the addition of essential oil of alpine pine are also health-giving for obese people.

Baths with a decoction of dried leaves and crushed roots of burdock are an effective remedy for obesity. In order to prepare the decoction, you need to take 30 g of dry vegetable mixture and to pour it with 1 liter of boiling water, to wrap it up, to let it infuse for 2 hours, to strain and to pour it into the bathtub. The bath temperature should be 36-37 °C. The course of treatment is 10-12 baths. These baths are recommended to be taken before bedtime.

Baths with nonherbal additives are used with good results. The simplest additive that turns an ordinary bath into therapeutic is salt.

Salt baths have a wide range of effects. They are indicated in diseases of the cardiovascular, nervous and musculoskeletal systems, in skin diseases. Salt bath helps at hyperexcitability, nervous exhaustion, allergies, improves health, has a rejuvenating effect on the body. The salt bath can also be used to combat obesity as the taking of such baths promotes excretion of decay products, toxins accumulated in it from overwork, as well as products, produced in the skin at its wilting. Salt baths are also indicated in arthritis, joint sprains and muscle injuries, diseases of women's reproductive system, cholecystitis. These baths are suitable for wound healing, ulcers or crust softening, which are the result of certain skin diseases. The peculiarity of such baths is the formation of so-called "salt cloak" (sediment of salt particles). It further irritates the receptors and nerve-endings, expanding blood vessels and stimulating blood circulation. The rush of heat during salt baths is one and a half times more intense than in fresh water. In addition, they have a soothing effect. Water bath should be 36-37 °C. The amount of salt may vary from one to several kilograms per bath. These baths are usually taken every other day, and the course of treatment consists of 12 to 15 baths. The course of treatment of these baths will depend on the desired effect. The treatment starts with a bath of pleasant temperature with a small amount of salt, gradually moving to more hot and concentrated ones. Salt baths are not suitable for very sensitive and delicate skin. It can successfully be replaced by a bath with mineral water (about mineral baths See below.).

Another traditional additive to make a therapeutic bath is starch. It has an enveloping, smoothing, antipruritic effect, protects sensitive skin from irritants. Therefore, starch baths are prescribed at skin diseases: neurodermatitis, ichthyosis, psoriasis, exudative child diathesis. These baths are prepared as follows: preliminarily dilute from 0.5 to 1 kg of starch in cold water, then, continuing to stir, add warm water and pour it into a bathtub; the water temperature should be 36-37 ° C. The duration of daily baths is 20-30 minutes. The course of treatment is 15-20 procedures. The treatment of children with starch bath is recommended to start no earlier than three years of age.

Baths with potassium permanganate have a disinfectant effect. They are recommended at pustular skin diseases, diaper rash. This is an effective bath with germicidal and drying effect. To prepare the bath, you need to dilute a few grains of potassium permanganate in 1 liter of water, to stir it thoroughly, making sure that all the grains are melted, and to pour into a water bath. The water must then be pale pink.

Turpentine baths became very popular In recent years. They are used to treat arthritis, any problems with vessels. A special emulsion is prepared for the baths. Dissolve 30 g of grated children soap in 550 ml of water, add 0.75 g of salicylic acid and simmer it, stirring with a wooden stick. Combine the hot mixture with 0.5 kg of pharmaceutic turpentine and stir it well. The emulsion is stored in tightly closed containers.

This emulsion is enough for 12-15 baths, baths are taken 2 days, taking a break on the third day. Bath duration is 15 minutes, the water temperature should be 37-38 °C, bath size – 150-170 liters. For the first 8 baths the emulsion is used in ascending order: 20, 30, ... 40 ml, for the remaining baths – 90 ml of the emulsion.

General recommendations for taking of mineral baths. It is known about the mineral water as a medical product for a long time. Two centuries ago it was very fashionable to spa among the well-off sectors of society – to drink and take mineral baths for recuperation and disease prevention. There are known some cases of treatment of certain diseases with mineral baths.

Mineral baths can be done at home, without leaving to the resort. Treatment should be carried out in courses. One such course should last from seven to ten days. Traditional healers prescribe the number of courses by the patient's state of health. If the illness lasts less than one year, then only one course is enough. If the disease is "old", the number of courses is equal to the number of years of the disease. Mineral water for prolonged use has a powerful all-round effect on the body, so it must be taken with caution and not to be misused. Bath with the addition of five to six liters of mineral water with gas stimulates tissue respiration, enriches the skin with oxygen, helps to relieve muscle spasm and relax. Both intake of mineral water as well as mineral bath lead to improved health.

Essential Oils Recipes

CHAPTER 10

Essential Oils for Baths

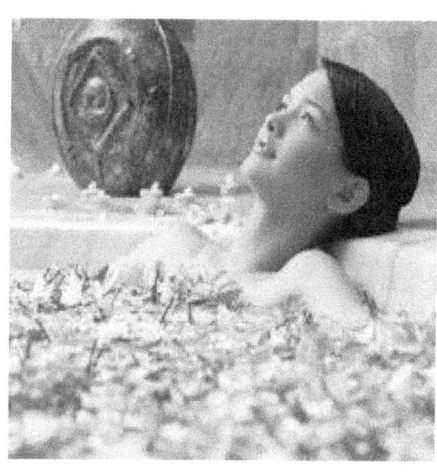

Use of essential oils for therapeutic baths

Recently, essential oils gained a great popularity. Baths with the addition of such oils may become an alternative of herbal mixtures. A few drops of oil should be added to the water in order to prepare an essential oil bath. The water temperature should be pleasantly warm in order to achieve a relaxing effect, to achieve a tonic effect – from slightly cool to cold. You don't need to take shower after taking a bath with oils. It is necessary to follow the recipe recommendations of the water temperature and selection of oils for therapeutic purposes.

Coconut oil is mainly for dry skin. It is necessary at frequent bathing as chlorinated water dries the skin greatly. In addition to adding the oil in the water bath, it can be applied to face skin and hair before taking a bath.

Avocado oil gently cleanses the pores and therefore suitable for sensitive skin. The oil is rich in vitamins, so it should be used rarely and in small doses, otherwise the opposite effect can occur, as an overdose of vitamin A can result in severe swelling.

Jojoba oil restores the natural level of the acid-base balance of the skin, promotes rapid healing of wounds, cuts.

Orange oil helps to maintain activity and cheerfulness at overstress, fatigue, during menopause, is effective for anti-aging skin care.

Jasmine oil is a natural anti-depressant. It has antiseptic, analgesic, sedative effect.

Lavender oil regulates the menstrual cycle and blood pressure. It helps at difficulties in the airways. For use as an additive to bath water, it dries the skin and treats acne well.

Lemon oil helps to relieve fatigue, slightly whitens skin.

Peppermint oil is an excellent antiseptic, used at cuts, irritation, itching, rubefaction. Relieves headaches.

Geranium oil helps at bad mood or depression; it is used to treat the common cold. Baths with geranium oil is highly recommended to people with weakened muscles and prone to fractures.

Juniper oil, added to the bath, will help with minor wounds and pustular skin diseases.

Hyssop oil is desirable to add to bath for meteodependent people, it reduces negative effects of changing weather patterns on the body.

Baths with the addition of rose oil give freshness and elasticity to the skin. They can be taken in any amount, there are no contraindications.

Baths with oil of all conifers improve blood flow of internal organs and skeletal muscles, eliminates pain. These baths are also indicated at bronchitis, rhinitis, neurasthenia, gastritis, menopausal disorders.

Hot bath with the addition of pine oil has a beneficial effect on the nervous system (especially for neurasthenia, neurosis, insomnia). Taking duration depends on the health and heart rate, but generally should not exceed 20 minutes.

The course of baths with essential oils is usually of 7-14 procedures. They are taken in a day, the duration of each bath is 10-

15 minutes. In order to prepare the bath, you need to add from 5 to 20 drops of essential oil. After several months the bath taking course can be repeated.

CHAPTER 11

Body Care at Home

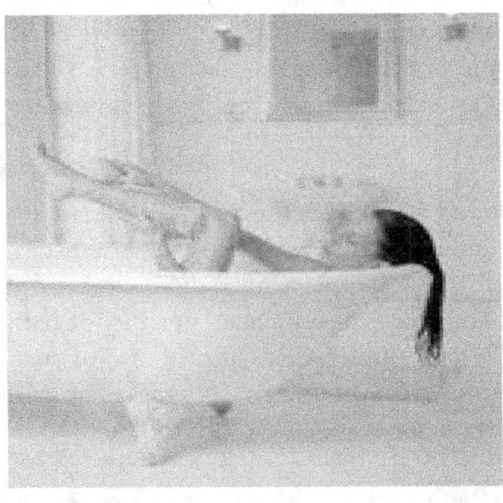

How to care for your legs skin at home.Useful tips and advice for women to care for their feet .

A pleasant procedure is very health-giving for your body a therapeutic bath.

Baths with sea salt or herbs are very health-giving. They calm the nervous system well, make you forget about the hassle, energize you and relieve fatigue.

Before you take a bath, it is necessary to wash yourself with a soap in a shower, so you open the pores and make the skin more susceptible to herbs effect. Now you can take a bath. Relax, take a comfortable position, all parts of your body must rest. The optimal time for taking a bath is 10-15 minutes. After the bath, your skin must be creamed or applied in body lotion, it can also be natural oils olive or sunflower. Apply them to your skin gently with circular movements. This procedure will leave a lasting feeling of freshness and renewal.

You can not only buy ready-made bath additives in a store, but you can also make them yourself (although, of course, you still have to buy some of the bath components, for example sea salt). We declare with confidence that your homemade bath additives will be no less effective than additives of factory manufacturing, packed in a beautiful boxes. Body skin becomes smooth, supple and healthy, as remedies, the recipes of which are listed below, have strong curative and restorative properties.

Real sea bath

You will need sea salt to it. Note that regular table salt is not suitable, because it does not contain minerals, which are in large amounts in sea salt. Sea salt is sold almost in any pharmacy and is not expensive, so it will be no problem for you to buy it.

Fill the bathtub with warm water and dissolve 400 g of sea salt in it. And now enjoy! The benefits of such a bath is very large: minerals, contained in sea salt, help to remove excess tissue fluid, making your skin smoother and pores tighter. In addition, sea bath is a good way to lose weight, especially when combined with other, more active methods of influence on extra weight.

Rose bath

You will need sea salt and rose petals for it. Take a kilo of sea salt and pour it into a jar, sprinkling each layer of salt with rose petals. The sea salt will fully absorb the rose fragrance after three weeks, and taking such bath will be a real pleasure for you. Such quantity of bath additives will be enough for a long time. Baths with the use of such remedy will be a real boon to you – a busy woman, who is up and running and maintains the household, and therefore difficultly cuts out free time for self-care.

Now immerse into a bath and soothe your taut nerves. Be sure: after taking such bath, you will feel yourself like a born again.

Citrus bath

If you love the smell of lemon, then this bath additive is just for you. Take 5-6 Tbsp. of dried lemon peel, chop it, brew in 1 liter of boiling water and leave to infuse for half an hour. Then the additive is ready: just pour it into a bathtub filled with warm water.

The effect, which this bath gives, is truly curative: first, toxins are derived from your body thanks to this great additive, which, of course, has a positive effect on the condition of your skin: it becomes more smooth and silky, gets a beautiful color. In addition, the bath, as well as coniferous one, has a soothing effect, allowing you to forget about household chores and problems, which all of us always have abound.

Soothing bath

It is recommended for a dry skin, prone to keratinization. Fill the bathtub with water of the body temperature and pour a very thick broth of oat flakes, add 2-3 Tbsp. of coniferous extract. Dry your skin with a towel and apply a cream with massage movements after the bath.

Coniferous bath

Pour the infusion of needles (1 cup for 2 liters of boiling water; infuse in a thermos for 2.5-3 hours) into the pre-prepared bath of just below the body temperature. It soothes, relaxes and relieves tension.

Aromatic bath

About an hour before taking a bath, prepare a decoction of dill, lavender, sage, rosemary, yarrow, chamomile (altogether it should be about 2 cups of mixed, chopped herbs). Pour the decoction into the water. Your skin will become fresh from this bath.

Cleopatra bath

Pour 2 liters of milk into a bathtub and add a cup of honey, oatmeal decoction. You won't recognize your skin. Oat decoction is done as follows. Pour 2 liters of water on a glass of raw oats (you can buy it at the market or the bird market, sold as food for birds), bring to the boil and cook for 15 minutes, cool, strain.

However, before you plunge into the warm fragrant bath, make sure that it serves your benefit, not harm. Yes, there are special rules for **taking a bath** which need to be strictly abided.

1.This bath shouldn't be taken very often (about once a week), otherwise you can earn serious circulatory disorders.

2.The temperature of the bath should be no more than 37 ° C.

3.Do not take a bath for longer than 15 minutes.

4.Be aware that these baths are not made to clean your skin, but to treat it and smooth, so there is no need in soaps and cleansers!

CHAPTER 12

Baths for Body. Recipes of Baths for Body

Baths for normal skin
Strawberry-birch bath
Required: 50 grams of dried leaves of birch and wild strawberries, 2 liters of water.

Preparation: Pour boiling water on the vegetative raw, leave it to infuse for an hour, strain, add to the bath with warm water.

Application: Take such bath once a week for 15-20 minutes.

Bath with hops
Required: 15-20 dried hop cones, 2 L of water.

Preparation: Pour boiling water on the hops, let it infuse for an hour, strain, add to the bath with warm water.

Application: Take such bath once a week for 15-20 minutes.
Tea bath
Required: 300 g of green and black tea, 2 L of water.

Preparation: Pour hot water on the vegetative raw, let it infuse for an hour, strain, add to the bath with warm water.

Application: Take such bath once a week for 10 minutes.

Milk and orange bath

Required: 2 L of cow's milk, 2 oranges.

Preparation: Squeeze the juice from oranges, heat the milk and mix it with the orange juice. Add the resulting mixture to the bath with warm water.

Application: Take such bath once a week for 15 minutes.

Milk and propolis bath

Required: 2 L of cow's milk, 50 g of propolis, honey.

Preparation: Heat the milk, add the propolis and the honey, mix thoroughly. Add the resulting mixture to the bath with warm water.

Application: Take such bath once a week for 15 minutes.

Honey-starch bath

Required: 200 g of honey, potato starch, 50 ml of 20% cream.

Preparation: Stir up the ingredients. Add the resulting mixture to the bath with very warm water.

Application: Take such bath once a week for 15 minutes.

Chamomile and lavender bath

Required: 50 grams of dried and chopped chamomile, lavender, 2 L of water.

Preparation: Pour hot water on the vegetative raw, let it infuse for an hour, strain, add to the bath with warm water.

Application: Take such bath once a week for 15-20 minutes.

Coniferous bath

Required: 3 handfuls of coniferous needles, 2 L of water.

Preparation: Pour hot water on the needles, let it infuse for 2 hours, strain, add to the bath with warm water.

Application: Take such bath once a week for 10 minutes.

Bath with thyme and yarrow

Required: 100 g of dried chopped yarrow, thyme, 2 L of water.

Preparation: Pour hot water on the vegetative raw, let it infuse for 1 hours, strain, add to the bath with warm water.

Application: Take such bath once a week for 15 minutes.

Watermelon bath

Required: 1 medium-sized watermelon, 0.5 L of milk.

Preparation: Squeeze the juice from watermelon pulp and mix with the milk. Pour the mixture into a bath with warm water.

Application: Take such bath once a week for 15 minutes.

Bath with henna and starch

Required: 100 g of a colorless henna and potato starch, 2 L of water.

Preparation: Pour hot water on henna, let it infuse for 30 minutes, strain, add starch to the infusion. Add the resulting mixture into the bath with very warm water.

Application: Take such bath once a week for 15 minutes.

Tea-coniferous bath

Required: 100 g of hibiscus tea, cedar needles, 2 L of water.

Preparation: Pour hot water on the vegetative raw, let it infuse for 2 hours, strain. Pour the infusion into the bath with warm water.

Application: Take such bath once a week for 10 minutes.

CHAPTER 13

Baths for Dry and Dehydrated Skin

Glycerin bath
Required:
200g of glycerin,
15 ml of lavenderoil.

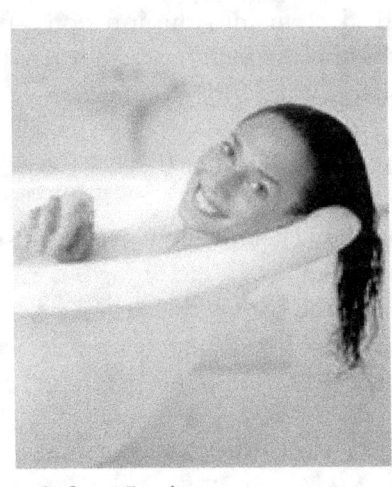

Preparation:
Stir the ingredients thoroughly, add to the bath with warm water.

Application: Take once a week for 15 minutes.

Simple Milk Bath

Required: 2 L of cow's milk.

Preparation: Heat the milk strongly, not bringing to a boil, then add in the bath with warm water.

Application: Take once a week for 15 minutes.

Milk and honey bath
Required: 2 L of cow's milk, 50 g of honey.

Preparation: Heat the milk, mix with honey. Add the resulting mixture to the bath with warm water.

Application: Take such bath once a week for 15 minutes.

Milk-oil bath

Required: 2 L of goat milk, 100 g of olive oil. *Preparation:* Heat the milk, add the oil, stir thoroughly. Add the resulting mixture to the bath with warm water.

Application: Take such bath once a week for 15 minutes.

Milk-fir bath

Required: 2 L of cow's milk, 5 ml of fir oil.

Preparation: Heat the milk, add the essential oil, stir thoroughly. Pour the resulting mixture into the bath of warm water.

Application: Take such bath once a week for 15 minutes.

Acetic-rose bath

Required: 200 ml of apple cider vinegar, 5 ml of rose oil.

Preparation: Mix the ingredients, add to the bath of warm water.

Application: Take such bath once a week for 10 minutes.

Glycerin-dandelion bath

Required: 100 g of dried chopped dandelion, 2 Tbsp. of glycerin, honey, 2 L of water.

Preparation: Pour hot water on the vegetative raw, let it infuse for an hour, strain. Add honey and glycerin into the infusion, stir thoroughly. Pour the resulting mixture into the bath of warm water.

Application: Take such bath once a week for 15 minutes.

Dandelion-milk bath

Required: 100 g of dried chopped dandelion, 0.5 L of cow's milk, 1.5 L of water.

Preparation: Pour hot water on the vegetative raw, let it infuse for an hour, strain. Add pre-warmed milk to the infusion, mix thoroughly. Add the resulting mixture to the bath with warm water.

Application: Take a bath once a week for 15 minutes.

Honey-glycerin bath *Required:* 100 g of honey, 2 Tbsp. of glycerin.

Preparation: Stir the ingredients thoroughly. Add the resulting mixture to the bath with warm water. *Application:* Take a bath once a week for 15 minutes.

Cedar-cream bath

Required: 200 ml of 20% cream, 10 drops of cedar oil, Tbsp. of propolis.

Preparation: Stir the ingredients thoroughly.

Add the resulting mixture to the bath with hot water.

Application: Take a bath once a week for 15 minutes.

Oat-milk bath

Required: 1 kg of oats, 0.5 L of goat milk, 1.5 L of water.

Preparation: Pour oat flakes into a gauze bag, put it in the water and cook for 15 minutes. Wring the bag. Pour the warm milk in the resulting broth. Add the resulting mixture to the bath with warm water. *Application:* Take a bath once a week for 15 minutes.

Potato and cucumber bath

Required: 5 cucumbers, potatoes, 10 drops of almond oil. *Preparation:* Wash the potatoes, do not peel them, squeeze the juice from the vegetables, mix with the essential oil. Add the resulting mixture to the bath with warm water.

Application: Take a bath once a week for 15 minutes.

Milk-Sage Bath

Required: 100 g of dried powdered herb of sage, 0.5 L of cow's milk, 1.5 L of water.

Preparation Pour hot water on the vegetative raw, let it infuse for an hour, strain. Add the pre-warmed milk to the infusion, stir thoroughly. Pour the resulting mixture into the bath with warm water.

Application: Take a bath once a week for 15 minutes. **Honey and olive bath**

Required: 100 g of honey, olive oil, 10 drops of ylang-ylang.

Preparation: Stir the ingredients thoroughly, add to the bath with hot water.

Application: Take such bath once a week for 10 minutes.

Castor-honey bath

Required: 20 ml of castor oil, 50 g of honey, 10 drops of rose oil.

Preparation: Mix the ingredients, heat and pour the resulting mixture into the bath with warm water.

Application: Take once in 2 weeks for 10 minutes.

Oil-cream bath

Required: 10 drops of fir and cedar oil, 100 ml of cream.

Preparation: Mix the ingredients, added to the bath with hot water.

Application: Take such bath once in 2 weeks for 10 minutes.

Cream-Milk Bath

Required: 1.5 L of milk, 100 ml of 20% cream, 5 g of shilajit.

Preparation: Heat the milk, dissolve shilajit in it, add the cream and stir thoroughly. Pour the resulting mixture into the bath with warm water.

Application: Take once a week for 10 minutes.

Acetic-**linden** bath

Required: 200 ml of apple cider vinegar, 100 grams of linden blossoms, 1 L of water.

Preparation: Pour hot water on the linden blossoms, let it infuse for 15 minutes, strain, add the vinegar. Pour the mixture into the bath with warm water.

Application: Take such bath once in 2 weeks for 10 minutes.

Acetic-laurel bath

Required: 200 ml of apple cider vinegar, 100 g of dried bay leaves, 1 L of water.

Preparation: Pour hot water on the bay leaves, let it infuse for 20 minutes, strain, add the vinegar. Pour the mixture into the bath with warm water.

Application: Take such bath once in 2 weeks for 10 minutes.

Acetic-juniper bath

Required: 200 g of crushed juniper branches, 50 ml of apple cider vinegar, 2 L of water.

Preparation: Pour hot water on the juniper, let it infuse for 20 minutes, strain, add the vinegar. Pour the mixture into the bath with warm water.

Application: Take such bath once in 2 weeks for 10 minutes.

CHAPTER 14

Baths for Sensitive and Irritated Skin

Bath with oak bark and mint
Required: 70 grams of powdered oak bark, 30 g of dried mint leaves, 2 L of water.
Preparation: Pour hot water on the vegetative raw, let it infuse for an hour, strain, add to the bath with warm water.
Application: Take such bath once a week for 15 -20 minutes.
Rose bath with milk
Required: 2 L of goat milk, 5 ml of rose oil, 5 g of the shilajit.
Preparation: Heat the milk, add the shilajit and oil to it, mix thoroughly.
Pour the resulting mixture into the bath with warm water.
Application: Take such bath once a week for 15 minutes.
Birch-**juniper** bath
Required: 100 g of crushed juniper branches, birch leaves, 2 L of water.
Preparation: Pour hot water on the vegetative raw, let it infuse for 2 hours, strain, pour into the bath with warm water
Application: Take once a week for 10 minutes.
Juniper-**oak** bath
Required: 100 g of crushed juniper branches, powdered oak bark, 2 L of water.

Preparation: Pour hot water on the vegetative raw, let it infuse for 2 hours, strain. Pour the infusion into the bath with warm water.

Application: Take once a week for 10 minutes.

Juniper-fir bath

Required: 100 g of crushed juniper and fir branches, 2 L of water.

Preparation: Pour hot water on the vegetative raw, let it infuse for 2 hours, strain. Pour the infusion into the bath with warm water.

Application: Take once a week for 10 minutes.

Juniper-walnut bath

Required: 100 g of crushed juniper branches, ground walnut leaves, 2 L of water.

Preparation: Pour hot water on the vegetative raw, let it infuse for 2 hours, strain. Pour the infusion into the bath with warm water.

Application: Take such bath once a week for 10 minutes.

Tea-juniper bath

Required: 100 grams of green tea, crushed juniper branches, 2 L of water.

Preparation: Pour hot water on the vegetative raw, let it infuse for 2 hours, strain. Pour the infusion into the bath with warm water.

Application: Take such bath once a week for 10 minutes.

Flax-juniper bath

Required: 100 grams of flaxseeds, crushed juniper branches, 2 L of water.

Preparation: Pour hot water on the vegetative raw, let it infuse for 2 hours, strain. Pour the infusion into the bath with warm water.

Application: Take such bath once a week for 10 minutes.

Dandelion and cotton thistle bath

Required: 100 g of dried chopped thistle, dandelion, 2 L of water.

Preparation: Pour hot water on the vegetative raw, let it infuse for 2 hours, strain. Add to the bath with warm water.

Application: Take such bath once a week for 15 minutes.

Bath with chamomile and celandine

Required: 30 g of dried chopped celandine, chamomile, 50 grams of propolis, 2 L of water.

Preparation Pour hot water on the vegetative raw, let it infuse for an hour, strain, heat, add the propolis and mix thoroughly. Add the resulting mixture to the bath with warm water.

Application: Take such bath once a week for 15 minutes.

Bath with oak bark and licorice

Required: 30 grams of dried powdered oak bark, licorice root, 1 handful of pine needles, 2 L of water.

Preparation: Pour hot water on the vegetative raw, let it infuse for an hour, strain. Pour the resulting infusion into the bath with warm water.

Application: Take once a week for 15 minutes.

Laurel and birch bath

Required: 100 g of powdered birch bark, colorless henna, 2 L of water.

Preparation: Pour hot water on the vegetative raw, let it infuse for an hour, strain. Pour the resulting infusion into the bath with warm water.

Application: Take such bath once a week for 10 minutes.

Tea and Birch Bath

Required: 100 grams of green tea, dried shredded birch buds, 2 L of water.

Preparation: Pour hot water on the vegetative raw, let it infuse for 2 hours, strain. Pour the infusion into the bath with warm water.

Application: Take such bath once a week for 15 minutes.

CONCLUSION

This book named **"Essential Oils and Aromatherapy for Weight Loss, Stress Relief and Happiness and fo Baths"** is a useful, as well as an interesting read for you, especially if you want to enhance your knowledge about the essential oils used for various treatments. In this book, it is unambiguously described that the essential oils are natural oils, which are different from fragrant oils. The applications of Aromatherapy are not confined to a massage room at the spa and thus, play a role in wellness. Now, it is not difficult at all to lose weight. Aromatherapy helps you in getting rid of the extra fat in your body. Aromatherapy is an easy way to lose weight via essential oils as compared to other ways, like diet control and strenuous exercise. A few essential oils are used in Aromatherapy to relieve you of the tension, anxiety and stress. Certain diseases related to stress can be cured via Aromatherapy. Last, but not the least, you can find your way to happiness via making these essential oils a part of your life. In this book, certain unique and useful recipes of the combination essential oils are given, which can prove to be real helpful for you!

This book is not intended as a substitute for the medical advice of physicians. The reader should regularly consult a physician in matters relating to his/her health and particularly with respect to any symptoms that may require diagnosis or medical attention.

www.ingramcontent.com/pod-product-compliance
Lightning Source LLC
Chambersburg PA
CBHW072119280526
45788CB00006B/2554